GLORIOUSTINA ESSIA

GREEN VIGOR

A MAN'S GUIDE TO HERBAL MEDICINE

Contents

INTRODUCTION

Embracing Herbal Wisdom for Men's Health

Welcome to "Green Vigor: A Man's Guide to Herbal Medicine," where the ancient art of herbal healing is unveiled to address the unique health concerns of men. In today's fast-paced world, where stress, processed foods, and sedentary lifestyles have become the norm, men's health faces numerous challenges. Yet, a powerful ally lies within plants' roots, leaves, and flowers for restoring balance, vitality, and wellness. Discover the natural pathways to optimal health, designed specifically for the male body and its unique requirements.

Often discussed in hushed tones or overlooked, men's health deserves attention and care. From the vitality of youth to the wisdom of age, every stage of a man's life brings its health concerns—prostate health, cardiovascular fitness, mental well-being, or physical strength. The modern approach to health, dominated by quick fixes and pharmaceutical interventions, often misses the holistic picture. Here, herbal medicine offers a more balanced, integrative approach to health that has been fine-tuned by centuries of traditional wisdom and modern research.

Embracing herbal wisdom for men's health is not about shunning modern medicine but complementing it with natural remedies that have stood the test of time. It's about taking charge of your health by understanding how various herbs can support your body's biological healing processes. This journey is as much about prevention as it is about healing, nurturing the body's inherent strengths, and addressing imbalances before they manifest into more significant health issues.

Herbs offer a gentle yet potent means to support the body, mind, and spirit. Whether using saw palmetto to support prostate health, harnessing the antioxidant power of hawthorn for heart health, or finding calm amid stress with the adaptogenic properties of ashwagandha, herbs provide a versatile toolkit for addressing a wide range of health concerns. However, embarking on this path requires more than knowledge of which herb to take; it requires understanding how to listen to your body and respond to its needs.

This guide to herbal wisdom for men's health is your starting point. It's an invitation to explore the natural world in a way that supports your health journey, offering insights into how to incorporate herbs into your daily life for optimal wellness. As you turn these pages, keep an open mind and heart. Be willing to experiment and learn from both the successes and the setbacks. Remember, the path to health is personal and ever-evolving.

As the 9th volume in the "Green Healing: The Natural Medicine Bible" series, "Green Vigor" builds upon the foundation of herbal knowledge in previous volumes, focusing on the unique aspects of men's health. It's a testament to the power of plants in supporting health and wellness and a guide to living a life in harmony with nature.

So, let's begin this journey together, exploring the ancient wisdom and modern science of herbal medicine. Let's embrace the plants around us, learning how they can support, heal, and nourish our bodies and minds. Welcome to a world where health is nurtured naturally, vitality springs from the very roots of the earth, and where every man has the tools to thrive. Welcome to "Green Vigor."

CHAPTER 1: THE HERBAL FOUNDATION FOR MEN

This chapter lays the groundwork for understanding how herbal medicine can be integrated into men's health and wellness strategies, emphasizing the importance of using herbs safely and effectively.

Understanding Herbal Medicine

Herbal medicine, known as phytotherapy, involves using plants' therapeutic properties to prevent and treat various health issues. For centuries, cultures around the globe have turned to the plant kingdom for healing, harnessing the natural compounds found in herbs to address a wide range of conditions. Today, this ancient practice is supported by a growing body of scientific research, affirming the efficacy of many traditional herbal remedies.

For men, herbal medicine offers a holistic approach to health, focusing on the body's natural healing abilities. It acknowledges that true wellness encompasses physical, mental, and emotional balance. Herbs like ginseng, known for its energy-boosting properties, or saw palmetto, used for prostate health, are just the tip of the iceberg. The world of herbal medicine is vast and varied, offering natural solutions for everything from cardiovascular health to stress management.

Safety Guidelines for Herbal Use

While herbs offer incredible health benefits, it's crucial to approach herbal medicine with mindfulness and respect. Here are some safety guidelines to ensure that your experience with herbal medicine is both positive and health-promoting:

- **Consult Healthcare Professionals:** Before adding any new herb to your regimen, especially if you have existing health conditions or are taking medication, consult a healthcare provider. Some herbs can interact with medications, potentially leading to adverse effects.
- **Quality Matters:** Source your herbs from reputable suppliers to ensure they are pure, high-quality, and contaminants-free. Organic and wild-crafted herbs are often preferred because they lack chemical pesticides and fertilizers.
- **Start Slow:** When trying a new herb, start with a lower dose to see how your body responds. Gradually adjust the dosage as needed, paying attention to changes in your body or health.
- **Educate Yourself:** Make an effort to learn about the herbs you're using. Understand their uses, benefits, and potential side effects. Knowledge is power, especially when it comes to your health.
- **Listen to Your Body:** Everyone's body reacts differently to herbs. What works for one person may only work for one person. Listen to your body and adjust your herbal regimen as needed. If you experience adverse effects, discontinue use and consult a healthcare provider.
- **Respect the Process:** Herbal medicine often works more subtly and slowly than conventional medicine. Give it time to see the full benefits, and remember that maintaining health is an ongoing process, not a one-time fix.

Herbal medicine opens up a world of natural healing possibilities, offering men a way to support their health holistically and preventatively. Understanding the basics of using herbs safely and effectively takes the first step toward a healthier, more balanced life. This chapter serves as your foundation in the vast and enriching field of herbal medicine, guiding you toward a deeper connection with the natural world and a more empowered approach to your health and well-being.

CHAPTER 2: HERBS FOR PROSTATE AND REPRODUCTIVE HEALTH

In the realm of men's health, the prostate and reproductive system hold significant importance, not just for physical well-being but also for a man's sense of vitality and wellness. Nature provides a treasure trove of herbs explicitly targeting these areas, offering support, healing, and enhancement. This chapter delves into how certain herbs like Saw Palmetto, Pygeum, Maca, and Ginseng play pivotal roles in nurturing prostate health, boosting fertility, enhancing libido, and addressing common reproductive issues naturally and holistically.

Nurturing the Prostate with Saw Palmetto and Pygeum

The prostate, a small gland pivotal for reproductive functions, can become a source of concern as men age, particularly with conditions like Benign Prostatic Hyperplasia (BPH). Nature offers remedies such as Saw Palmetto and Pygeum, which have been studied for their beneficial effects on prostate health.

- **Saw Palmetto (Serenoa repens):** Rich in fatty acids and phytosterols, Saw Palmetto is renowned for effectively reducing urinary symptoms associated with an enlarged prostate. Its mechanism involves the inhibition of DHT (a hormone that contributes to prostate growth), offering relief and support for those with BPH.

- **Pygeum (Prunus africana):** Derived from the bark of the African cherry tree, Pygeum is another herb known for its prostate health benefits. It reduces inflammation and promotes healthy urination patterns, making it a valuable ally in managing BPH symptoms.

Incorporating these herbs into your wellness routine can provide supportive care for your prostate. Still, it's essential to consult with a healthcare provider, especially if you're experiencing significant symptoms or are on medication.

Enhancing Fertility and Libido: The Role of Maca and Ginseng

Fertility and a healthy libido are often reflections of overall health and vitality. Maca and Ginseng stand out for their long history of use in enhancing reproductive health and sexual vitality.

- **Maca (Lepidium meyenii):** This Peruvian root is famed for boosting libido and improving sexual function without affecting hormone levels directly. It's also revered for increasing energy, stamina, and endurance, contributing to its reputation as a natural aphrodisiac.
- **Ginseng (Panax ginseng):** Often called the "king of herbs," Ginseng is acclaimed for enhancing vitality and sexual health. Studies suggest that it can improve erectile function, sexual desire, and overall energy levels, making it a cornerstone herb for men's reproductive health.

A Herbal Approach to Preventing and Addressing Common Reproductive Issues

Beyond the proactive nurturing of the prostate and enhancing fertility, herbal medicine offers solutions for a range of reproductive issues, from erectile dysfunction to hormonal imbalances.

- **Tribulus Terrestris:** Known for its libido-enhancing properties, Tribulus can also support sperm health and testosterone levels, offering a multi-faceted approach to male reproductive wellness.
- **Ashwagandha (Withania somnifera):** This adaptogen doesn't just combat stress; it's also shown promise in improving semen quality and hormonal balance, underlining the interconnectedness of stress, fertility, and overall health.

CHAPTER 3: SUPPORTING CARDIOVASCULAR HEALTH WITH HERBS

In the quest for a healthy heart and robust cardiovascular system, herbs offer a beacon of hope and a testament to the power of nature's pharmacy. The modern lifestyle, characterized by high stress, sedentary habits, and processed foods, greatly strains heart health. Yet, amidst this, the ancient wisdom of herbal medicine provides natural allies like Hawthorn and Garlic, along with other botanicals, to support and protect our cardiovascular system.

Hawthorn and Garlic: Allies for a Healthy Heart

The heart, our most vital organ, requires nourishment and care to function optimally. Hawthorn and Garlic stand out for their exceptional cardiovascular benefits, backed by centuries of use and contemporary research.

- **Hawthorn (Crataegus spp.):** Revered for its heart-protective properties, Hawthorn enhances heart muscle function, increases blood flow, and helps regulate blood pressure. Its rich flavonoid content is the key to its efficacy, offering antioxidant protection and improving overall cardiac health. Incorporating Hawthorn into your regimen, whether through teas, tinctures, or capsules, can provide foundational support for heart health.
- **Garlic (Allium sativum):** Beyond its culinary acclaim, Garlic is a power-house for cardiovascular wellness. Its ability to lower blood pressure,

reduce cholesterol levels, and inhibit platelet aggregation makes it a valuable tool in preventing arterial plaque buildup. Fresh Garlic, aged extracts, or supplements can be used to harness these benefits, making Garlic a versatile and potent ally for heart health.

Managing Blood Pressure Naturally

High blood pressure, or hypertension, is a silent threat that significantly increases the risk of heart disease and stroke. Nature offers a bounty of herbs that can help manage blood pressure naturally.

- **Celery Seed (Apium graveolens):** This humble spice has shown promise in reducing blood pressure thanks to its diuretic and vasodilatory effects. Used in culinary dishes or taken as a supplement, Celery Seed can be a simple yet effective addition to a heart-healthy lifestyle.
- **Hibiscus (Hibiscus sabdariffa):** The vibrant Hibiscus flower, steeped as a tea, has been shown to lower blood pressure in several studies. Its tart, cranberry-like flavor makes it a refreshing choice for daily consumption.

Herbs for Cholesterol Management and Circulatory Support

Managing cholesterol levels is crucial for cardiovascular health, preventing the buildup of plaque that can lead to heart disease. Herbs offer natural solutions to support this balance.

- **Red Yeast Rice (Monascus purpureus):** Used in Traditional Chinese Medicine, Red Yeast Rice contains compounds similar to statin drugs, which can help lower LDL (harmful) cholesterol levels. It's essential to use this under the guidance of a healthcare professional due to its potent effects and potential interactions.
- **Ginkgo Biloba:** Known for enhancing circulatory health, Ginkgo Biloba improves blood flow to the brain and extremities, supporting overall

vascular health. It mainly benefits older adults, preventing circulatory diseases and cognitive decline.

Embracing herbs for cardiovascular health is about creating a holistic balance where natural remedies complement healthy lifestyle choices. Hawthorn, Garlic, Celery Seed, Hibiscus, Red Yeast Rice, and Ginkgo Biloba are examples of how the plant kingdom supports heart health. Integrating these herbs into your daily routine, alongside a balanced diet, regular exercise, and stress management practices, can significantly improve cardiovascular wellness. Remember, the journey to heart health is a marathon, not a sprint. It requires patience, consistency, and a deep commitment to nurturing your body with nature's gifts.

CHAPTER 4: HERBS FOR MUSCLE AND JOINT HEALTH

Muscle and joint health is fundamental to maintaining an active, fulfilling life. Whether you're an athlete, someone who enjoys a weekend hike, or someone navigating the natural challenges of aging, the wear and tear on your muscles and joints can significantly impact your quality of life. Fortunately, nature provides us with a bounty of herbs like Arnica, Comfrey, Turmeric, and Ginger, each with powerful properties to soothe discomfort, reduce inflammation, and support the body's healing processes.

Relief for Sore Muscles: Arnica and Comfrey

After physical activity, sore muscles are a common complaint, often signaling overuse or the natural process of strength building. However, relief doesn't always have to come from a pill bottle.

- **Arnica (Arnica montana):** Renowned for reducing pain and inflammation, Arnica is a go-to herb for athletes and fitness enthusiasts. Applied topically as a cream, gel, or salve, Arnica helps alleviate muscle soreness and reduce bruising, making it an essential component of any natural first-aid kit. Note that Arnica should not be applied to broken skin or taken internally unless in a homeopathic formulation.
- **Comfrey (Symphytum officinale):** With a long history of use for healing sprains, strains, and broken bones, Comfrey is known as the "knitbone"

herb. Its active compound, allantoin, promotes the growth of new cells, thereby accelerating healing. Comfrey creams and poultices can be applied directly to sore muscles, offering relief and speeding recovery. Due to its potent effects, Comfrey should be used with care, and it's advisable not to apply it to open wounds or use it for extended periods.

Natural Solutions for Joint Pain: Turmeric and Ginger

Joint pain, often due to inflammation, can severely limit mobility and diminish life quality. Turmeric and Ginger, celebrated for their anti-inflammatory properties, offer natural pathways to relief.

- **Turmeric (Curcuma longa):** The golden spice Turmeric, rich in curcumin, stands out for its potent anti-inflammatory and antioxidant properties. Incorporating Turmeric into your diet or taking it as a supplement can help alleviate joint pain and stiffness associated with conditions like arthritis. For enhanced absorption, pair Turmeric with black pepper, which contains piperine, significantly increasing curcumin's bioavailability.
- **Ginger (Zingiber officinale):** Like Turmeric, Ginger is a powerful anti-inflammatory herb that can reduce pain and improve mobility in osteoarthritis and rheumatoid arthritis. Ginger can be consumed fresh, dried, or as a supplement, making it a versatile and effective remedy for joint pain.

Strengthening Connective Tissues with Herbal Remedies

Beyond addressing pain and inflammation, nurturing the health of connective tissues is vital for long-term joint health.

- **Horsetail (Equisetum arvense):** Rich in silica, Horsetail helps form collagen, an essential building block of bones, cartilage, and other connective tissues. Taking Horsetail as a tea or supplement can support the structural integrity of joints and improve their overall health.

- **Gotu Kola (Centella Asiatica):** Gotu Kola promotes the health of connective tissues by stimulating collagen production and supporting circulatory health. This herb is particularly beneficial in healing wounds and improving skin elasticity, with implications for joint health by supporting the surrounding structures.

The journey toward maintaining and improving muscle and joint health is multifaceted, encompassing exercise and nutrition and the strategic use of herbal remedies. Arnica, Comfrey, Turmeric, Ginger, Horsetail, and Gotu Kola each offer unique benefits that can soothe discomfort, reduce inflammation, and strengthen the body's support structures.

CHAPTER 5: STRESS RELIEF AND MENTAL HEALTH FOR MEN

In today's fast-paced world, the mental health and well-being of men often take a backseat to the demands of life, work, and societal expectations. Stress, anxiety, and mood fluctuations are not just challenges to overcome but opportunities to nurture more profound resilience and balance. With its array of adaptogens, natural mood boosters, and calming herbs, the plant kingdom offers a treasure trove of remedies to support men's mental health. This chapter explores how Ashwagandha, Rhodiola, St. John's Wort, Lemon Balm, Valerian, and Passionflower can be integrated into daily routines to foster tranquility, uplift spirits, and improve sleep.

Adaptogens for Stress Management

Adaptogens are a unique class of herbs known for their ability to help the body resist and adapt to physical, chemical, or biological stress.

- **Ashwagandha (Withania somnifera):** Often called Indian Ginseng, Ashwagandha has been used for centuries in Ayurvedic medicine to enhance vitality and combat stress. Its ability to lower cortisol levels makes it invaluable for men dealing with chronic stress, promoting a sense of calm and well-being. Incorporating Ashwagandha into your diet, through capsules or powder mixed into smoothies, can help modulate the body's stress response, supporting overall mental health and resilience.

- **Rhodiola (Rhodiola rosea):** Rhodiola is celebrated for its energy-boosting and fatigue-reducing properties. Rhodiola can enhance focus, stamina, and mood by balancing the stress hormone cortisol. It is an excellent herb for men facing high-pressure environments or those looking to improve their mental performance and endurance.

Natural Mood Boosters

The natural world is rich in herbs that can lift the mood and bring light to darker days, acting as gentle yet effective mood boosters.

- **St. John's Wort (Hypericum perforatum):** This herb is well-known for its antidepressant properties, offering support for mild to moderate depression. St. John's Wort increases neurotransmitters such as serotonin and dopamine in the brain, contributing to a more positive mood and emotional balance. Caution is advised due to its potential interactions with certain medications.
- **Lemon Balm (Melissa officinalis):** With its refreshing lemon scent, Lemon Balm is a beautiful herb for alleviating anxiety and elevating mood. Its mild sedative effect can reduce stress without causing drowsiness, making it perfect for daytime use. Lemon Balm tea is a delightful way to incorporate this herb into your routine, offering a moment of calm and joy amidst the hustle of daily life.

Herbs for Sleep and Anxiety

Quality sleep is foundational to mental health, yet many men struggle with insomnia and anxiety that can disrupt restful nights. Valerian and Passionflower are two herbs that can help ease the mind and promote better sleep.

- **Valerian (Valeriana officinalis):** Valerian root has been used for centuries to treat insomnia and promote relaxation. By enhancing GABA (a neurotransmitter that helps regulate nerve impulses in your brain and nervous system) levels in the brain, Valerian helps ease anxiety and encourages deep, restorative sleep.

- **Passionflower (Passiflora incarnata):** This flowering plant treats anxiety and sleep disorders effectively. Its calming properties help quiet the mind, making it easier to fall asleep and stay asleep through the night. Passionflower can be taken as a tea, tincture, or capsule, making it a versatile addition to your evening routine.

The journey toward improved mental health and stress relief is deeply personal. While herbs offer profound support, they do so most effectively within the context of a holistic approach to wellness. Incorporating adaptogens, mood boosters, and sleep aids like Ashwagandha, Rhodiola, St. John's Wort, Lemon Balm, Valerian, and Passionflower into your life can open the door to enhanced mental resilience, emotional balance, and overall well-being. Embrace these herbal allies with mindfulness, and let them guide you to a place of strength and tranquility in mind and spirit.

CHAPTER 6: ENHANCING VITALITY AND ENERGY WITH HERBS

For men seeking to elevate their physical performance and endurance or infuse their daily routine with a boost of natural energy, herbs like Ginseng and Cordyceps stand out.

The Energizing Power of Ginseng and Cordyceps

- **Ginseng (Panax ginseng):** Ginseng is often hailed as the ultimate tonic for vitality. It is revered in traditional medicine for enhancing energy levels, improving stamina, and supporting recovery after exertion. Its adaptogenic properties make it particularly beneficial for combating fatigue, as it helps the body adapt to stress and enhances overall energy metabolism. Incorporating Ginseng into your daily regimen can be as simple as starting your morning with a Ginseng tea or taking a Ginseng supplement, providing a sustained energy boost without the jitters associated with caffeine.

- **Cordyceps (Cordyceps Sinensis):** This unique fungus, found growing on the larvae of caterpillars in the high mountains of China, has gained popularity for its ability to increase ATP production (the primary energy carrier in cells). This increase in ATP means improved oxygen utilization and cellular energy, translating to enhanced physical performance and endurance. Cordyceps can be consumed in powdered form, added to smoothies, or taken as a supplement, making it a versatile option for those looking to elevate their energy levels naturally.

Herbs for Endurance and Physical Performance

Beyond the immediate boost of energy, sustaining endurance and enhancing physical performance is crucial for athletes and active individuals.

- **Rhodiola (Rhodiola rosea):** Another potent adaptogen, Rhodiola, is known for improving endurance and resilience to physical and mental stress. By enhancing oxygen transport and reducing recovery time, Rhodiola is ideal for those engaging in high-intensity activities or seeking to push their physical boundaries.
- **Beetroot (Beta vulgaris):** While not an herb in the traditional sense, Beetroot deserves mention for its high nitrate content, which the body converts into nitric oxide. This process improves blood flow and oxygen delivery to muscles, significantly enhancing endurance and physical performance. Beetroot juice or powder can easily be incorporated into pre-workout routines for a natural performance boost.

Balancing Hormones and Boosting Vitality Naturally

At the core of vitality and energy lies the hormonal balance. Several herbs are known for supporting hormonal health and, by extension, enhancing vitality.

- **Ashwagandha (Withania somnifera):** By modulating the stress hormone cortisol, Ashwagandha helps manage stress and supports the balance of testosterone, an essential hormone in men's health. This balancing act can improve energy, muscle strength, and overall vitality.
- **Tribulus Terrestris:** Often used to support libido, Tribulus also balances hormones and enhances vitality. IncreasingIncreasing luteinizing hormone levels signals the body to produce more testosterone naturally, supporting energy, performance, and muscle development.

The journey to enhanced vitality and energy is multifaceted, intertwining diet, exercise, rest, and the strategic use of herbs. Ginseng, Cordyceps, Rhodiola, Beetroot, Ashwagandha, and Tribulus Terrestris each offer unique benefits that support the body's natural energy production, improve endurance, and contribute to hormonal balance. By incorporating these natural powerhouses into your wellness routine, you can embrace a life filled with vigor and vitality. Remember, the key to harnessing the full potential of these herbs lies in listening to your body, consulting with healthcare professionals, and committing to a holistic approach to health and well-being.

CHAPTER 7: INTEGRATING HERBS INTO DAILY LIFE

Embracing herbal medicine is a journey toward natural wellness that invites a deeper connection with nature's rhythms and our bodies' wisdom. As we explore how herbs can enhance our health, vitality, and well-being, we must consider how these powerful allies can seamlessly integrate into our daily lives. This chapter is dedicated to crafting your herbal toolkit, offering lifestyle tips for maximizing the benefits of herbs, and guiding you in building a personalized herbal wellness plan.

Crafting Your Herbal Toolkit: Teas, Tinctures, and Supplements

- **Teas:** Herbal teas are perhaps the most accessible and enjoyable way to incorporate herbs into your routine. Whether it's a calming cup of chamomile before bed, a midday energizing brew of green tea, or a soothing sip of peppermint to aid digestion, teas offer a simple method to enjoy the benefits of herbs. Experiment with single herbs or blend them to create custom mixtures that cater to your health needs and taste preferences.
- **Tinctures** are concentrated herbal extracts from soaking herbs in alcohol or vinegar. They provide a potent and convenient way to consume herbs, especially on the go. A few drops of tincture can be added to water or tea or taken directly under the tongue for quick absorption. Tinctures are

particularly useful for herbs that aren't as palatable as teas or when you require a more concentrated dose.

- **Supplements:** For those who prefer convenience or need specific, consistent dosages of an herb, supplements in the form of capsules or tablets can be a practical option. When choosing supplements, look for reputable brands that provide transparency about sourcing and extraction methods to ensure you get the highest quality product.

Lifestyle Tips for Maximizing Herbal Benefits

- **Consistency is Key:** Consistency matters when using herbs, like any aspect of health and wellness. Regularly incorporating them into your routine enhances their efficacy, allowing your body to adjust and respond to their benefits.
- **Listen to Your Body:** How your body reacts to different herbs. What works wonderfully for one person may have a different effect on another. If an herb doesn't agree with you, don't hesitate to try alternatives that might be more compatible with your body's unique needs.
- **Educate Yourself:** Understanding herbs' properties, uses, and potential interactions will empower you to choose which ones to include in your wellness plan. Continuously seek reliable information and consider consulting with a herbalist or healthcare provider to deepen your herbal knowledge.

Building a Personalized Herbal Wellness Plan

Creating a personalized herbal wellness plan involves assessing your health goals, current lifestyle, and any specific challenges or conditions you face. Identify areas you'd like to improve, such as stress management, sleep quality, energy levels, or specific health concerns. From there, research herbs that align with your goals and consider how to incorporate them into your daily routine, whether through teas, tinctures, supplements, or culinary uses.

Remember to start slowly, introducing one herb at a time to monitor its effects before adding more. This approach helps you understand how individual herbs impact your well-being and reduces the risk of potential interactions. As you grow more comfortable and knowledgeable, you can begin experimenting with combining herbs for synergistic effects.

Integrating herbs into daily life is a practice of mindfulness, intention, and connection to the natural world. It's a journey that invites patience, curiosity, and a willingness to engage actively in your path to wellness. You embark on a profoundly rewarding path toward holistic health by crafting your herbal toolkit, embracing lifestyle practices that enhance the benefits of herbs, and building a personalized plan. Let the wisdom of herbs guide you, nurture you, and inspire you toward a life of vitality and harmony.

CHAPTER 8: ADVANCED HERBAL THERAPIES FOR MEN

Embarking on a journey toward optimal health involves addressing immediate concerns, focusing on preventative measures, enhancing longevity, and maintaining cognitive strength. Advanced herbal therapies offer men a path to achieve these goals naturally. This chapter explores sophisticated herbal strategies focusing on detoxification, anti-aging, and cognitive enhancement, aiming to provide a holistic approach to men's health beyond the basics.

Detoxification and Cleansing Herbs

In our modern environment, exposure to toxins, whether from pollution, processed foods, or chemical products, is almost inevitable. A periodic detox can help eliminate these toxins, supporting the body's natural cleansing processes and enhancing overall well-being.

- **Milk Thistle (Silybum marianum):** Renowned for its liver-protective qualities, it supports the liver in its critical detoxification role. The active compound, silymarin, not only aids in eliminating toxins but also has regenerative properties, helping to repair liver cells damaged by exposure to harmful substances.

- **Dandelion (Taraxacum officinale):** Dandelion's root and leaves are powerful detoxifying agents. Dandelion stimulates digestion, aids the kidneys in filtering out waste, and supports liver function. Incorporating

Dandelion tea or supplements can gently promote detoxification and internal cleansing.

- **Burdock Root (Arctium lappa):** Burdock Root is another herb that supports detoxification through its blood-purifying and diuretic properties. It helps to eliminate toxins through increased urination and promotes overall skin health, often reflecting the body's internal state.

Longevity and Anti-Aging Herbs

The quest for longevity and a life full of vitality is as old as humanity itself. Certain herbs have been identified for their remarkable anti-aging properties, supporting a longer, healthier life.

- **Ginseng (Panax ginseng):** Ginseng is the most well-known herb for promoting longevity. Its adaptogenic properties help the body resist stress, while its antioxidant effects combat free radical damage, a critical factor in aging.
- **Ginkgo Biloba:** Ginkgo is celebrated for enhancing circulation and protecting neurological health. Ginkgo Biloba supports cognitive function well into old age by improving blood flow to the brain and acting as an antioxidant.
- **Astragalus (Astragalus membranaceus):** Used in Traditional Chinese Medicine to bolster the immune system and prevent disease, Astragalus is associated with increased lifespan and anti-aging effects. Its compounds may help protect telomeres, the caps at the end of each strand of DNA, from degradation.

Herbs for Cognitive Enhancement and Focus

Maintaining cognitive agility and focus is essential for accomplishing daily tasks and sustaining mental health. Several herbs can enhance cognitive function, memory, and concentration.

- **Bacopa Monnieri:** Bacopa, a traditional Ayurvedic herb, is revered for its cognitive-enhancing properties. Studies suggest it improves memory, attention, and the ability to process visual information, making it an excellent herb for mental clarity and focus.
- **Rhodiola Rosea:** By reducing mental fatigue and improving resilience to stress, Rhodiola can significantly enhance focus and productivity. Its adaptogenic qualities make it particularly beneficial during intense mental work or study.
- **Lion's Mane Mushroom (Hericium erinaceus):** The Lion's Mane is a unique mushroom known for its neuroprotective properties. It stimulates the production of nerve growth factors, aiding in the maintenance and growth of neurons, thereby supporting cognitive function and mental acuity.

Advanced herbal therapies offer a promising avenue for men seeking to detoxify their bodies, enhance longevity, and maintain sharp cognitive functions. By incorporating these herbs into a holistic health regimen that includes a balanced diet, regular exercise, and stress management techniques, men can significantly improve their quality of life and overall well-being.

CHAPTER 9: RECIPES AND REMEDIES FOR MEN'S HEALTH

Navigating the path to optimal health requires more than just knowledge—it demands action. This chapter translates the wisdom of herbal medicine into practical, DIY formulations and remedies specifically tailored to men's health concerns. From daily tonics that invigorate vitality to specific remedies addressing common health issues, these herbal solutions empower men to take proactive steps towards their well-being with nature's bounty.

DIY Herbal Formulations for Everyday Use

Daily Vitality Tonic:

A robust tonic that supports overall vitality, immune function, and stress resilience, perfect for daily consumption.

- **Ingredients:**
- 1 part Ashwagandha root
- 1 part Ginseng (Panax ginseng) root
- 1/2 part Ginkgo Biloba leaves
- Honey or maple syrup to taste
- 4 cups of water
- **Instructions:**

1. Combine the Ashwagandha, Ginseng, and Ginkgo Biloba with water in a saucepan.
2. Bring to a boil, then simmer on low heat for 30 minutes.
3. Strain the mixture and add honey or maple syrup to sweeten.
4. Drink a small cup each morning to kickstart your day with natural energy.

Muscle Recovery Salve:

Ideal for soothing sore muscles after workouts, this salve uses the healing properties of Arnica and Comfrey.

- **Ingredients:**
- 2 tablespoons Arnica flowers
- 2 tablespoons Comfrey leaves
- 1/2 cup Coconut oil
- 1/4 cup Beeswax pellets
- **Instructions:**

1. Infuse Arnica flowers, and Comfrey goes in coconut oil over low heat for 2-3 hours. Avoid boiling.
2. Strain the herbs from the oil using cheesecloth.
3. Return the infused oil to the saucepan, add beeswax pellets, and heat until melted.
4. Pour the mixture into a jar or tin and let it solidify.
5. Apply to sore muscles as needed, taking care to avoid broken skin.

Energizing Morning Tea Blend

Kickstart your day with a blend that boosts energy without the jitteriness of caffeine.

- **Ingredients:**
- 1 part Green Tea leaves

- 1 part Yerba Mate leaves
- ½ part Ginseng root (finely chopped)
- ½ part Peppermint leaves
- **Instructions:**

1. Mix all the herbs and store them in an airtight container.
2. To make the tea, steep 1 teaspoon of the blend in 1 cup of hot water for 5-7 minutes.
3. Strain and enjoy in the morning to energize your day.

Stress-Busting Herbal Tincture

This tincture is perfect for men dealing with daily stress and looking for a natural way to unwind.

- **Ingredients:**
- 1 part Ashwagandha root
- 1 part Holy Basil leaves
- 1 part Skullcap leaves
- Vodka or apple cider vinegar
- **Instructions:**

1. Fill a jar one-third of the way with the mixed dried herbs.
2. Pour vodka or vinegar over the herbs until wholly submerged.
3. Seal the jar and store it in a cool, dark place for 4-6 weeks, shaking it daily.
4. After steeping, strain the tincture through cheesecloth and store it in dropper bottles.
5. Take 1-2 droppers full under the tongue or in water when you need stress relief.

Immune-Boosting Herbal Syrup

Support your immune system with this potent, delicious syrup, which is especially beneficial during cold and flu seasons.

- **Ingredients:**
- 1 part Echinacea root
- 1 part Elderberry
- ½ part Ginger root
- ¼ part Cinnamon bark
- Honey
- Water
- **Instructions:**

1. Combine all the herbs in a pot (1 cup of water for every tablespoon).
2. Bring to a boil, then simmer until the liquid is reduced by half.
3. Strain the herbs, and mix in an equal part of honey while the liquid is still warm (not hot).
4. Bottle the syrup and take 1 tablespoon daily for immune support or every few hours at the first sign of illness.

Post-Workout Muscle Recovery Oil

Soothe sore muscles and accelerate recovery with this infused oil, ideal after intense workouts or physical activity.

- **Ingredients:**
- 1 part Arnica flowers
- 1 part St. John's Wort
- Olive or sweet almond oil
- **Instructions:**

1. Fill a jar with the dried herbs and cover entirely with oil.

2. Place the jar in a warm, sunny spot for 4 weeks, shaking daily.

3. Strain the oil through cheesecloth and store it in a clean bottle.

4. Massage the oil into sore muscles as needed, avoiding broken skin.

Bedtime Sleep Aid Tea

Encourage deep, restorative sleep with this calming herbal tea blend.

- **Ingredients:**
- 1 part Chamomile flowers
- 1 part Valerian root
- 1 part Lavender flowers
- ½ part Lemon Balm leaves
- **Instructions:**

1. Combine all the herbs and store them in an airtight container.

2. To prepare the tea, steep 1 teaspoon of the blend in 1 cup of hot water for 10 minutes.

3. Drink 30 minutes before bedtime to promote a peaceful night's sleep.

Mental Clarity and Focus Blend

This herbal tea blend boosts cognitive function and concentration, perfect for morning or midday slumps.

- **Ingredients:**
- 1 part Ginkgo Biloba leaves
- 1 part of Gotu Kola leaves
- ½ part Rosemary leaves
- ½ part Peppermint leaves
- **Instructions:**

1. Mix all the herbs in an airtight container.

2. To prepare the tea, steep 1 teaspoon of the blend in 1 cup of hot water for about 10 minutes.

3. Strain and enjoy when you need mental clarity and focus.

Soothing Aftershave Lotion

Calm and rejuvenate your skin post-shave with this natural, herbal-infused lotion.

- **Ingredients:**
- ¼ cup Witch Hazel
- ¼ cup Aloe Vera gel
- 2 tablespoons Calendula-infused oil
- 10 drops of Lavender essential oil
- 5 drops of Tea Tree essential oil
- **Instructions:**

1. Combine all ingredients in a bottle and shake well to mix.
2. Apply to your face and neck to soothe and moisturize the skin after shaving.

Digestive Bitters Tonic

Stimulate digestion and improve gut health with this homemade bitters tonic, ideal before meals.

- **Ingredients:**
- 1 part Dandelion root
- 1 part Burdock root
- 1 part Fennel seeds
- ½ part Ginger root
- Vodka or apple cider vinegar
- **Instructions:**

1. Fill a jar with the mixed dried herbs.
2. Cover entirely with vodka or vinegar.
3. Seal the jar and let it sit in a cool, dark place for 4 weeks, shaking it daily.
4. Strain the liquid and take a teaspoon before meals to aid digestion.

Respiratory Health Syrup

Support and clear your respiratory pathways with this herbal syrup, which is especially useful during cold and allergy seasons.

- **Ingredients:**
- 1 part Mullein leaves
- 1 part Elecampane root
- ½ part Licorice root
- ¼ part Peppermint leaves
- Honey
- Water
- **Instructions:**

1. Simmer the herbs in water until the liquid is reduced by half.
2. Strain the herbs and mix the remaining liquid with an equal part of honey.
3. Bottle the syrup and take 1 teaspoon up to three times daily for respiratory support.

Daily Energy Support Tincture

Maintain steady energy levels throughout the day without the crash associated with caffeine.

- **Ingredients:**
- 1 part Eleuthero root (Siberian Ginseng)
- 1 part Schisandra berries
- ½ part Rhodiola root

- Vodka or apple cider vinegar
- **Instructions:**

1. Combine the herbs in a jar and cover them with vodka or vinegar.
2. Seal the jar and let it sit for 4 weeks, shaking it daily.
3. Strain and store in dropper bottles. Take 1-2 droppers full of water or juice in the morning or early afternoon for an energy boost.

Specific Remedies for Men's Health Concerns

Prostate Health Tea:

A supportive tea blend for maintaining prostate health, featuring the synergistic effects of Saw Palmetto and Nettle.

- **Ingredients:**
- 1 teaspoon Saw Palmetto berries (crushed)
- 1 teaspoon Nettle leaves
- Honey to taste
- 1 cup of boiling water
- **Instructions:**

1. Place Saw Palmetto berries and Nettle leaves in a tea infuser or pot.
2. Pour boiling water over the herbs and steep for 10-15 minutes.
3. Strain (if necessary) and add honey to taste.
4. Enjoy once daily to support prostate health.

Stress Relief Adaptogen Blend:

A calming tincture blend featuring adaptogens like Rhodiola and Ashwagandha, designed to mitigate stress and enhance mental clarity.

- **Ingredients:**

- 1 part Rhodiola root
- 1 part Ashwagandha root
- Vodka or apple cider vinegar
- **Instructions:**

1. Fill a jar 1/3 full with dried Rhodiola and Ashwagandha roots.
2. Pour vodka or apple cider vinegar over the herbs until wholly submerged.
3. Seal the jar and store it in a cool, dark place, shaking daily for 4-6 weeks.
4. Strain the tincture through cheesecloth and store it in amber dropper bottles.
5. Take 1-2 droppers full to combat stress and support adrenal health.

Cardiovascular Support Tea

A heart-healthy tea blend that supports circulation and cardiovascular health.

- **Ingredients:**
- 1 part Hawthorn berries
- 1 part Hibiscus flowers
- ½ part Ginkgo Biloba leaves
- ½ part Nettle leaves
- **Instructions:**

1. Mix all the herbs in an airtight container.
2. To brew, steep 1 tablespoon of the blend in 1 cup of boiling water for 10-15 minutes.
3. Drink daily to support heart health and circulation.

Prostate Wellness Tincture

A tincture blend aimed at supporting prostate health and urinary function.

- **Ingredients:**

- 1 part Saw Palmetto berries
- 1 part Nettle root
- ½ part Pumpkin seeds
- Vodka or apple cider vinegar
- **Instructions:**

1. Coarsely grind or crush the herbs and seeds, then place them in a jar.
2. Cover the herbal mixture with vodka or vinegar, completely submerging the herbs.
3. Seal the jar and let it sit in a cool, dark place for 4-6 weeks, shaking it daily.
4. Strain the liquid and store it in amber dropper bottles. Take 1-2 droppers complete daily or as directed by a healthcare provider.

Anti-stress and Anxiety Herbal Capsules

Capsules filled with a blend of adaptogenic herbs to mitigate stress and promote mental calmness.

- **Ingredients:**
- Ashwagandha powder
- Rhodiola Rosea powder
- Holy Basil (Tulsi) powder
- **Instructions:**

1. In a bowl, mix equal parts of each powdered herb thoroughly.
2. Fill empty capsules with the blend using a capsule machine or a small spoon.
3. Take 1-2 capsules to combat stress and support adrenal health.

Joint and Muscle Relief Salve

A soothing topical salve for relieving joint pain and muscle aches.

- **Ingredients:**
- ¼ cup Arnica flower-infused oil
- ¼ cup St. John's Wort-infused oil
- 2 tablespoons Beeswax
- 10 drops Peppermint essential oil
- 10 drops Eucalyptus essential oil
- **Instructions:**

1. Gently heat the infused oils and beeswax in a double boiler until the beeswax is melted.
2. Remove from heat and stir in the essential oils.
3. Pour the mixture into small tins or jars and let cool until solidified.
4. Apply to sore muscles and joints as needed for relief.

Sleep Enhancing Herbal Pillow

Create an herbal pillow to promote restful sleep, filled with herbs known for calming and sleep-inducing properties.

- **Ingredients:**
- Dried Lavender flowers
- Dried Chamomile flowers
- Dried Lemon Balm leaves
- A small cloth bag or pillow
- **Instructions:**

1. Mix equal parts of dried Lavender, Chamomile, and Lemon Balm.
2. Fill the cloth bag or pillow with the herbal mixture and seal it.
3. Place the herbal pillow near your head or under your pillow at night to

inhale the calming scents and promote restful sleep.

Mental Alertness Boosting Tincture

This tincture is formulated to enhance focus, memory, and cognitive function throughout the day.

- **Ingredients:**
- 1 part Bacopa (Bacopa monnieri)
- 1 part Ginkgo Biloba
- 1 part Rosemary (Rosmarinus officinalis)
- Alcohol (vodka or grain alcohol) for extraction
- **Instructions:**

1. Combine the herbs in a glass jar and cover them with alcohol, completely submerging them.
2. Seal the jar and place it in a cool, dark place. Shake daily for 4-6 weeks.
3. Strain the mixture into a clean bottle using a fine mesh strainer or cheesecloth.
4. Use 1-2 droppers of the tincture in water or juice in the morning or early afternoon to enhance mental clarity and focus.

Skin Health Herbal Oil

An infused oil nourishes the skin, promotes healing, and prevents acne and irritation. It is perfect for after shaving.

- **Ingredients:**
- 1 part Calendula (Calendula officinalis)
- 1 part Plantain leaf (Plantago major)
- Olive oil or sweet almond oil for infusion
- **Instructions:**

1. Fill a jar with dried Calendula and Plantain leaves, then pour the oil over the herbs until fully covered.
2. Seal the jar and place it in a sunny window for 4 weeks, shaking occasionally.
3. Strain the infused oil into a clean bottle.
4. Apply to the skin as needed, especially after shaving, to soothe, heal, and moisturize.

Digestive Support Herbal Blend

A blend to support digestion, relieve bloating, and enhance nutrient absorption.

- **Ingredients:**
- 1 part Peppermint (Mentha piperita)
- 1 part Fennel seeds (Foeniculum vulgare)
- 1 part Ginger root (Zingiber officinale)
- **Instructions:**

1. Mix the herbs and store them in an airtight container.
2. Steep 1 teaspoon of this blend in a cup of boiling water for 10 minutes.
3. Drink after meals to aid digestion and relieve discomfort.

Respiratory Health Steam Inhalation

A herbal steam to clear congestion, support respiratory health and soothe irritation from colds or allergies.

- **Ingredients:**
- 1 part Eucalyptus leaves (Eucalyptus globulus)
- 1 part Thyme (Thymus vulgaris)
- 1 part Peppermint (Mentha piperita)
- **Instructions:**

1. Boil a pot of water and remove it from the heat.
2. Add a handful of the mixed herbs to the hot water.
3. Drape a towel over your head and lean over the pot, inhaling the steam for 5-10 minutes.
4. Perform once or twice daily to help clear the airways and ease breathing.

Energy-Boosting Herbal Snack Balls

Nutrient-dense, herbal-infused snack balls for a quick energy boost during the day.

- **Ingredients:**
- 1 cup dates, pitted
- ½ cup nuts (almonds, walnuts, or a mix)
- 2 tablespoons Maca powder
- 1 tablespoon Cacao powder
- 1 tablespoon Coconut oil
- Shredded coconut or cacao nibs for coating
- **Instructions:**

1. Blend the dates and nuts in a food processor until they form a sticky mixture.
2. Add the Maca powder, Cacao powder, and Coconut oil, blending until the mixture is well combined.
3. Roll the mixture into small balls, then coat with shredded coconut or cacao nibs.
4. Store in the refrigerator and consume one or two balls when you need an energy boost.

The journey to health and wellness is deeply personal, and integrating herbal remedies into your daily routine can offer profound benefits. These DIY formulations and specific treatments for men's health concerns are designed to empower you to harness the healing power of herbs in a practical, effective manner. As you experiment with these recipes, remember to listen to your body and adjust as needed. The path to wellness is iterative, a process of learning and growth. With these herbal allies by your side, you're well-equipped to navigate this journey with confidence and a deep connection to the natural world.

CONCLUSION

A Sustainable Path to Wellness: Embodying the Principles of Herbal Medicine

As we close this exploration into the rich world of herbal medicine tailored for men, we're reminded that true wellness transcends the mere absence of disease. It's a harmonious state where physical health, mental clarity, and emotional well-being are balanced. Embracing herbal medicine isn't just about utilizing plants for their healing properties; it's about adopting a sustainable approach to health that respects the body's natural rhythms, the environment, and the interconnectedness of all life.

Embracing a Holistic View

Herbal medicine teaches us to view health holistically, recognizing that every aspect of our lives contributes to our well-being. This perspective encourages us to treat symptoms and explore and address the root causes of health issues. It invites us to look beyond the physical and consider how our emotions, thoughts, environment, and lifestyle choices impact our health. In doing so, we begin to see ourselves as part of a larger ecosystem, where each element influences and is influenced by the others.

Learning from Nature

Nature operates on principles of balance and sustainability, constantly adapting to maintain harmony. By aligning ourselves with these principles, we can foster resilience and adaptability in our own lives. Herbs, with their adaptogenic qualities, offer us a model for thriving amid stress and change. They remind us of the importance of flexibility, bending rather than breaking under pressure. As we incorporate herbs into our wellness routines, we do more than ingest their active compounds; we imbibe nature's wisdom, learning to live sustainably and sustainably.

A Commitment to Self-Care

Adopting herbal medicine as part of our approach to health is ultimately an act of self-care. It's a commitment to nurturing ourselves, preparing a nourishing herbal tea, researching and understanding our herbs, and listening to our bodies with compassion and attentiveness. This self-care extends beyond the individual to the planet itself, as choosing sustainably sourced herbs and supporting ecological agriculture practices contribute to the health of the Earth.

The Journey Continues

The path to wellness is not a destination but a unique journey for each individual. It's a journey marked by learning, growth, and discovery, where each step brings us closer to understanding ourselves and the natural world. Embodying the principles of herbal medicine means embracing this journey with an open heart and mind, ready to explore the vast potential for healing within and around us.

As you move forward, let the principles of herbal medicine guide you on your path to wellness. Remember that balance, sustainability, and a holistic perspective are keys to a healthy life. Let the herbs be your allies, nature your teacher, and your well-being your most cherished goal. In doing so, you'll enhance your life and contribute to the world's more excellent health and harmony. This is the essence of a sustainable path to wellness—living in a way that nourishes you today and ensures the well-being of future generations.

APPENDICES

Embarking on the herbal medicine journey equips us with powerful tools for enhancing health and wellness. However, with great power comes great responsibility. To harness the full potential of herbal remedies while ensuring safety and efficacy, we must approach herbal medicine with knowledge, respect, and caution. This concluding section provides essential guidelines for safe herbal usage, suggests resources for further learning, and offers a glossary of common herbs and their uses, aiming to support and enrich your herbal wellness journey.

Herb Safety and Dosage Guidelines

Understanding Dosage:

Dosage can vary widely depending on the herb, the form in which it's consumed (tea, tincture, capsule, etc.), and the individual taking it. Start with the lowest recommended dose and consider your body's response. Consulting a professional herbalist or healthcare provider can provide personalized dosage advice.

Quality Matters:

Always source herbs from reputable suppliers. Organic and sustainably wildcrafted herbs are preferable to minimize pesticide exposure and support ecological health.

Herb-Drug Interactions:

Some herbs can interact with prescription medications, enhancing or inhibiting their effects. If you take any medications, consult a healthcare provider before adding new herbs.

Side Effects:

While herbs are generally safe, they can cause side effects or allergic reactions in some individuals. Discontinue use if you experience adverse reactions and seek professional advice.

Special Populations:

Pregnant or nursing women, children, and those with pre-existing health conditions should exercise caution with herbal remedies. Some herbs may not be suitable for these groups.

Glossary of Herbs and Their Uses

Ashwagandha (Withania somnifera):
  Adaptogen that helps manage stress and improve energy levels.
  Chamomile (Matricaria recutita): Soothes digestion and promotes relaxation and sleep.
  Echinacea (Echinacea spp.): Boosts the immune system and combats colds and flu.
  Ginger (Zingiber officinale): Stimulates digestion, relieves nausea, and has anti-inflammatory properties.
  Lavender (Lavandula angustifolia): Reduces anxiety and stress and promotes sleep.
  Milk Thistle (Silybum marianum): Supports liver health and detoxification.
  Nettle (Urtica dioica): Rich in nutrients; supports joint health, allergy relief, and urinary function.

Turmeric (Curcuma longa): Contains curcumin, known for its anti-inflammatory and antioxidant effects.

Valerian (Valeriana officinalis): Promotes relaxation and sleep, helping with insomnia and anxiety.

SOURCES

https://blog.mountainroseherbs.com/building-a-herbal-starter-kit

https://www.healthline.com/health/enlarged-prostate/natural-remedies

https://www.verywellhealth.com/herbs-for-an-enlarged-prostate-89389

https://www.clevelandheartlab.com/blog/top-herbs-for-your-heart/

https://www.gaiaherbs.com/blogs/seeds-of-knowledge/herbs-to-help-support-a-healthy-and-happy-heart

https://www.medicalnewstoday.com/articles/325760

https://www.detoxify.com/blogs/health/9-sacred-herbs-for-a-whole-body-detox

https://www.avogel.co.uk/health/muscles-joints/5-top-herbs-for-muscle-and-joint-pain/

https://www.canyonranch.com/well-stated/post/5-herbs-and-spices-for-natural-detoxification/

https://www.shantitea.ca/home/blog_article/st/85474/top-10-detoxifying-herbs

https://www.healthline.com/nutrition/16-ways-relieve-stress-anxiety

https://www.verywellmind.com/best-herbs-and-spices-for-brain-health-4047818

https://www.webmd.com/balance/features/natural-brain-boosters

https://guardian.ng/life/5-herbs-for-memory-boost-and-concentration/

https://www.pukkaherbs.com/uk/en/wellbeing-articles/plant-power-to-help-memory-and-stress

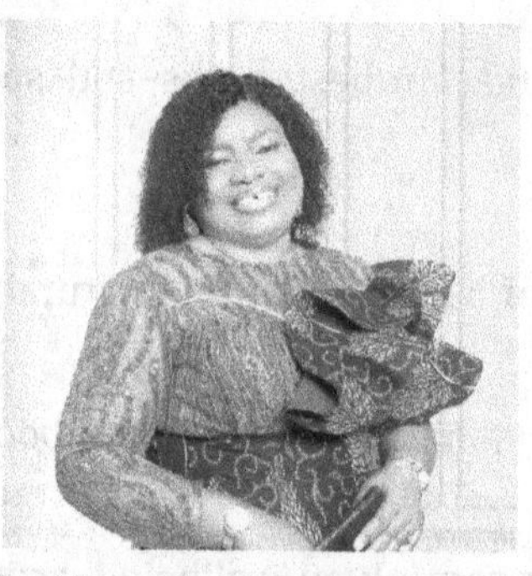

About the Author

Glorioustina Essia is a multifaceted professional whose expertise traverses the realms of technology, artificial intelligence, literature, and natural health. As a driving force in artificial intelligence, particularly in prompt engineering, she has established herself as a pioneer. Her proficiency extends to project management, network marketing, website development, and copywriting, showcasing a unique blend of technical understanding and creative flair.

A prolific author and publisher, Glorioustina's literary works span multiple genres, captivating a diverse audience with her narrative skill and inspiring a new generation of writers to unlock their creative potential. Her passion for storytelling matches her commitment to exploring and advocating for holistic health practices. Renowned in herbal medicine, she dedicates her life to studying and promoting natural health.

Glorioustina Essia's professional and personal journey is characterized by an unwavering dedication to her core strengths and a ceaseless pursuit of knowledge. Her zeal and expertise embody the limitless possibilities that arise from a commitment to innovation, quality, and a deep-seated passion for understanding the future of technology and the ancient wisdom of herbal medicine. Glorioustina is a testament to the power of interdisciplinary knowledge and its impact in a world where technology, literature, and natural health converge.

You can connect with me on:

🌐 https://www.amazon.com/author/glorioustina

Also by Glorioustina Essia

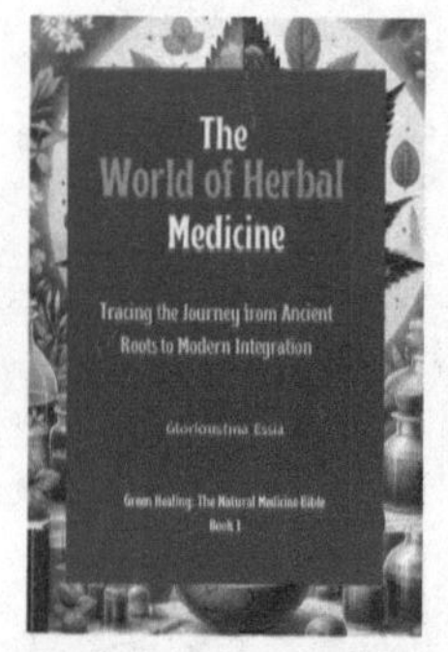

The World of Herbal Medicine

In an era where the rush of modern medicine often overshadows the pursuit of holistic health, the timeless wisdom of herbal remedies remains largely untapped. Do you find yourself seeking a more natural approach to health and wellness yet still determining where to begin or how to integrate these practices with modern healthcare?

Embark on a transformative journey with Book 1 of "Green Healing: The Natural Medicine Bible": "The World of Herbal Medicine." This enlightening volume takes you through the ancient pathways to the modern integration of herbal healing. Discover herbal medicine's rich history and evolution across different cultures, including the profound insights of Traditional Chinese Medicine, Ayurveda, and indigenous practices. Unravel how herbalism has evolved through historical epochs and how it beautifully intersects with modern medical practices today.

Embrace the journey to holistic health – add this captivating volume to your collection and begin exploring the world of herbal medicine today!

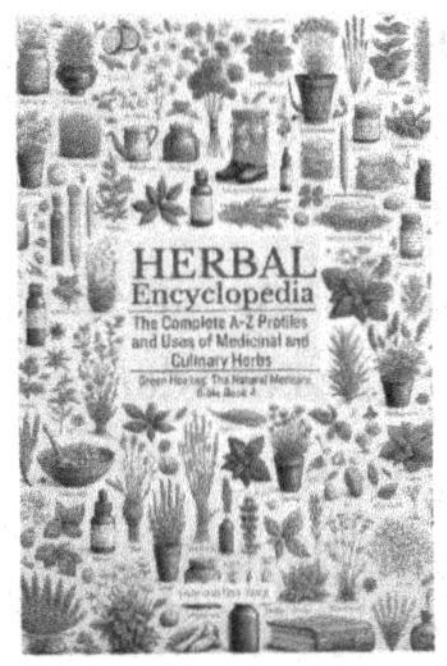

Herbal Encyclopedia

Embark on a journey through nature's apothecary with "Herbal Encyclopedia: The Complete A-Z Profiles and Uses of Medicinal and Culinary Herbs." This guide unravels the secrets of herbs, from age-old medicinal uses to enhancing culinary delights. Each page introduces you to a new herb, revealing its history, health benefits, and how it can be incorporated into your daily life. Whether you're a budding herbalist or a seasoned enthusiast, this encyclopedia offers easy-to-understand profiles, practical tips, and a connection to the ancient art of herbal healing.

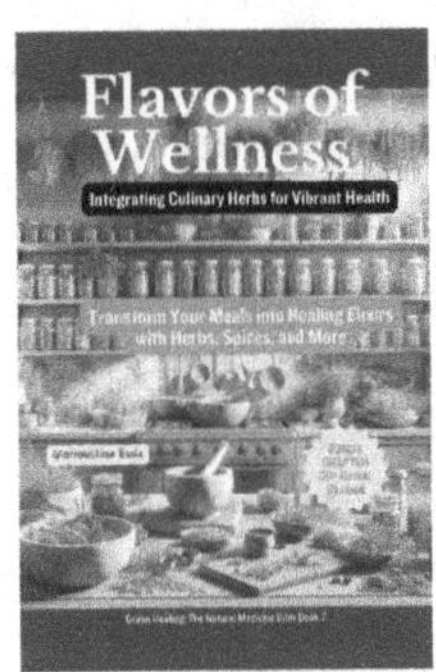

Flavors of Wellness

This guide invites you into a world where every herb in your garden or kitchen pantry is a key to unlocking vibrant health and elevating your culinary creations. From basil-infused breakfasts to rosemary-laced dinners, discover how to weave the magic of herbs into everyday cooking. Learn to grow, harvest, and preserve your herbs, ensuring your dishes burst with flavor and nutritional benefits all year round. Whether you're a novice cook or a seasoned chef, this book offers simple, delicious ways to incorporate healing herbs into your daily diet. Embrace the herbal lifestyle—where wellness and flavor live harmoniously on your plate.

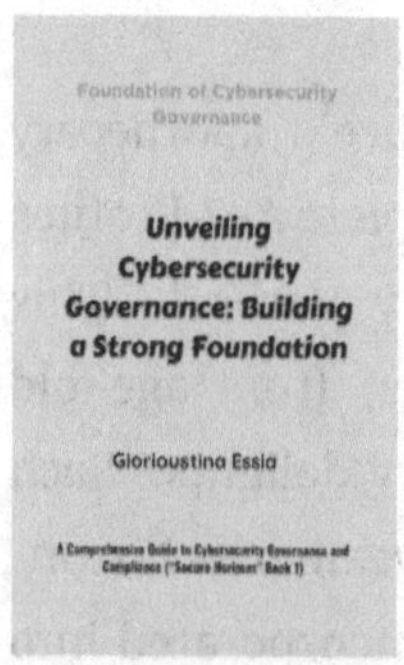

Unveiling Cybersecurity Governance

In the ever-expanding digital landscape, safeguarding sensitive information and maintaining robust cybersecurity practices have become paramount. "Unveiling Cybersecurity Governance: Building a Strong Foundation" is a comprehensive guide that delves into cybersecurity governance's core principles and components, equipping readers with the knowledge and tools to establish a secure digital environment.

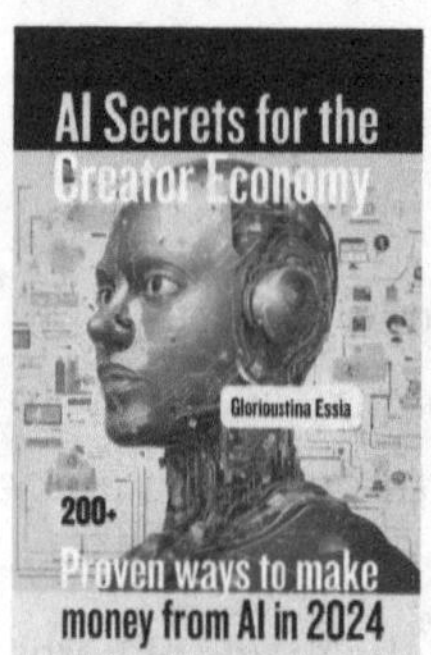

AI Secrets for the Creator Economy: 200+ Proven ways to make money from AI in 2024

In a world driven by innovation and transformation, the Creator Economy emerges as a powerful force, with Artificial Intelligence (AI) at its beating heart. This book, "AI Secrets for the Creator Economy: 200+ Proven Ways to Make Money from AI in 2024 and Beyond," is more than just a book; it's your key to unlocking the incredible synergy between AI and creativity, opening the door to a wealth of opportunities for those who are willing to seize them.

www.ingramcontent.com/pod-product-compliance
Lightning Source LLC
Chambersburg PA
CBHW012311240726

48656CB00008B/2639